The Amazing Ketogenic Cookbook for Beginners

Healthy and Tasty Ketogenic Recipes to Boost Your Diet and Enjoy Your Meals

I0145913

Lauren Loose

Contents

Pesto Zoodles..8

Low Carb BBQ Sauce 10

Tzatziki 12

Satay Sauce...14

Thousand Island Salad Dressing 16

Hollandaise Sauce..18

Taco Flavored Cheddar Crisps.......................................20

Ketogenic Seed Crispy Crackers....................................22

Scrambled Eggs with Mushrooms and Cheese 24

Peanut Butter Chocolate Smoothie 25

Cream Cheese Pancakes 26

Coconut Chia Pudding..27

Morning Hash 28

Spanish Scramble..29

Cheese Waffles..30

Spinach Frittata...31

Ketogenic Oatmeal...33

Baked Eggs 34

Blueberry Smoothie...35

Quick Ketogenic Pancakes 36

Spinach Quiche..38

Cream Crepes 40

Smoothie Bowl...42

Almond Butter Muffins...43

Classic Western Omelet...45

Sheet Pan Omelet..47

Detoxifying Green Smoothie 48

Nutty Pumpkin Smoothie..49

Salmon-Avocado Breakfast Boats 50

Buffalo Blue Cheese Omelet...51

Bacon, Egg & Cheese   Fat Bombs................................53

Cheesy Scrambled   Eggs & Greens 55

Mocha-Coconut Chia Pudding..57

Pumpkin Muffins..59

Almond Flour Pancakes 61

Warm Grain-Free Cereal 63

Corned Beef Hash and Eggs 65

Spiced Pear Breakfast Bars..67

Scrambled Eggs with   Buttered Basil.......................69

Breakfast Bake...70

Nutty Granola...72

Nutty Blueberry Muffins 74

Low-Carb Pancakes..76

Avocado and Eggs 78

Mushroom Frittata 80

Artichoke Omelet 82

Low-Carb Crepe...84

Cinnamon Almond Butter Smoothie.............................85

Kale Wrapped Eggs 86

Zucchini Ketogenic Bread 88

Ham Sausage Quiche 90

Coconut Almond Breakfast 92

Avocado Egg Muffins 94

Soft-Boiled Eggs 96

Breakfast Casserole 98

Poblano Cheese Frittata 101

Poached Egg 103

Spinach Egg Bites 105

Bacon Cheeseburger Waffles 107

Ketogenic Breakfast Cheesecake 110

Pesto Zoodles

Preparation time: 10 minutes

Cooking time: 10 minutes

Servings: 4 servings

Ingredients:

2 cups of new basil leaves

1 garlic clove, crushed.

1/3 cup of pine nuts

3 tablespoons of ground Parmesan cheddar

1/3 cup of extra-virgin olive oil, or a variant

Salt and newly ground dark pepper

1 tablespoon of extra-virgin olive oil

1 sweet onion daintily cut.

4 zucchinis cut into noodles (utilizing a device like this)

Parmesan cheddar twists, for garnishing

Red-pepper pieces, for decorating (discretionary)

Directions:

Make the Pesto: In a food processor or blender, beat the basil, garlic, pine nuts, and ground Parmesan until coarsely slashed.

With the food processor running, include the olive oil gradually and blend until the pesto is thick like glue. Add progressively the olive oil varying to alter the consistency. Add pepper and salt.

Make the Zoodles: In a large sauté container, heat the oil over medium warmth. Include the onion and sauté until delicate, or for 4 to 5 minutes. Include the zucchini noodles and sauté until delicate, or for 4 to 5 minutes more.

Include the pesto and stir until the noodles are very much covered.

Serve warm, decorated with Parmesan twists and red-pepper pieces, if used to taste.

Nutrition:

Calories: 422

Total Fat: 36.3g

Cholesterol: 0mg

Sodium: 201mg

Total Carbs: 24.4g

Fiber: 3.9g

Sugars: 5g

Protein: 6.5g

Low Carb BBQ Sauce

Preparation time: 10 minutes

Cooking time: 5 minutes

Servings: 1-16 ounces

Ingredients:

1/4 cup of Lecanto Gold dark colored sugar substitute OR sugar of your choice

1/4 cup of apple juice vinegar

1/4 cup of white vinegar

1/2 cup of water

2 tablespoons of genuine spread

1 would tomato be able to glue.

1 teaspoon of garlic powder

1 teaspoon of onion powder

1 teaspoon of dry yellow mustard

1 teaspoon of salt

1 teaspoon of cayenne pepper (discretionary)

1 teaspoon of fluid smoke (discretionary)

Directions:

If you like a thinner sauce, add more water until desired thickness is achieved.

If you like an increasingly acrid sauce, add more vinegar.

Go simple with the fluid smoke, a little is enough!

This formula is effectively versatile to various sugars. Utilizing a white sugar will bring about a sauce that is increasingly red in color.

The margarine makes a pleasant lustrous completion and makes the sauce to be on whatever you brush it on.

Nutrition:

Calories: 35

Total Fat: 0.4g

Cholesterol: 0mg

Sodium: 1198mg

Total Carbs: 5.9g

Fiber: 1.4g

Sugars: 3g

Protein: 1.3g

Tzatziki

Preparation time: 10 minutes

Cooking time: 0 minutes

Servings: 8 servings

Ingredients:

½ c shredded cucumber, drained.

1 tsp. salt

1 T olive oil

1 T fresh mint finely chopped.

2 garlic cloves

1 c full-fat Greek yogurt

1 t lemon juice

Directions:

Place shredded cucumber on a strainer for an hour or squeeze out moisture through a cheesecloth.

Mix all ingredients in a medium bowl.

Refrigerate.

Use as a vegetable dip, a dip for dehydrated vegetables, or a sauce for lamb, beef, or chicken. It is also a perfect accompaniment for fried summer squash.

Nutrition:

Calories: 79

Carbohydrates: 3g

Protein: 1g

Fat: 7g

Satay Sauce

Preparation time: 10 minutes

Cooking time: 15 minutes

Servings: 4 servings

Ingredients:

1 can (14 oz.) coconut cream (if you cannot find coconut cream, coconut milk works well)

1 dry red pepper, seeds removed, chopped fine.

1 clove garlic, minced.

¼ cup gluten-free soy sauce

1⊡3 c natural unsweetened peanut butter

salt and pepper

Directions:

Place all ingredients in a small saucepan. Bring the mixture to a boil.

Stir while heating to mix peanut butter with other ingredients as it melts.

After the mixture boils, turn down the heat to simmer on low heat for 5 to 10 minutes.

Remove from heat when the sauce is at the desired consistency. Adjust seasoning to taste.

This is a good sauce for chicken or turkey. Just add the sauce during the last minutes of baking or grilling. It can also be used as a dipping sauce.

Nutrition:

Calories: 312

Carbohydrates: 7g

Protein: 7g

Fat: 30g

Thousand Island Salad Dressing

Preparation time: 5 minutes

Cooking time: 5 minutes

Servings: 8 servings

Ingredients:

2 Tbs. olive oil

¼ c frozen spinach, thawed.

2 T dried parsley

1 T dried dill

1 t onion powder

½ t salt

¼ t black pepper

1 c full-fat mayonnaise

¼ c full-fat sour cream

Directions:

Combine all ingredients in a small mixing bowl.

Nutrition:

Calories: 312

Carbohydrates: 2g

Protein: 1g

Fat: 34g

Hollandaise Sauce

Preparation time: 10 minutes

Cooking time: 15 minutes

Servings: 4 servings

Ingredients:

4 egg yolks

2 T lemon juice

1 ½ sticks of butter, melted.

Salt and pepper

Directions:

Heat water to boil in a saucepan.

Separate the eggs. Save the whites for another use.

Place the yolks in a heat-resistant bowl, either glass or stainless steel.

Carefully melt the butter in a saucepan without burning.

Place the bowl with the egg yolks over the simmering water to gently heat the eggs. Make sure the water is not touching the bottom of the bowl. The eggs need to be steamed, not cooked.

Add lemon juice to egg yolks.

Slowly stream the melted butter into the egg yolks while whisking. Start with a few drops of butter and then add a slow stream. Whisk the eggs the entire time until all the butter is added, and the sauce has thickened.

Season to taste with lemon juice, salt, and pepper; you can also add a dash of Tabasco sauce.

Serve over poached eggs or cooked vegetables.

Nutrition:

Calories: 566

Carbohydrates: 1g

Protein: 3g

Fat: 62g

Taco Flavored Cheddar Crisps

Preparation time: 5 minutes

Cooking time: 10 minutes

Servings: 6 servings

Ingredients:

¾ c sharp cheddar cheese, finely shredded

¼ c parmesan cheese, finely shredded

¼ t chili powder

¼ t ground cumin

Directions:

Preheat the oven to 400 degrees.

Line cookie sheet with parchment paper

In a bowl, toss all ingredients together until well mixed.

Make 12 piles of cheese parchment paper.

Press down the cheese into a thin layer of cheese.

Bake for 5 minutes until cheese if bubby.

Allow to cool on parchment paper.

When completely cool, peel the paper away from the crisps.

These are a good Ketogenic substitute for chips. They are cheesy and crisp. Enjoy!

Nutrition:

Calories: 63

Fat: 5g

Sodium: 102mg

Total Carbs: 0.5g

Fiber: 0.1g

Sugars: 0.1g

Protein: 4g

Ketogenic Seed Crispy Crackers

Preparation time: 10 minutes

Cooking time: 45 minutes

Servings: 30 servings of 1 cracker

Ingredients:

1⧠ cup almond flour

1⧠ cup sunflower seed kernels

1⧠ cup pumpkin seed kernels

1⧠ cup flaxseed

1⧠ cup chia seeds

1 tbsp. ground psyllium husk powder

1 tsp. salt

¼ cup melted coconut oil.

1 cup boiling water.

Directions:

Preheat the oven to 300 degrees.

Stir all dry ingredients together in a medium-sized bowl until thoroughly mixed.

Add coconut oil and boiling water to dry ingredients and stir until all ingredients are mixed well.

On a flat surface, roll the dough between two pieces of parchment paper until approximately ⅛ inch thick.

Slide the dough, still between parchment papers onto a baking sheet.

Remove the top layer of parchment paper and place dough on a baking sheet into the oven.

Bake 40 minutes until golden brown.

Score the top of the dough into cracker sized pieces.

Leave in the oven to cool down.

When the big cracker is cool, break into pieces.

These crackers can be stored in an airtight container after they are completely cool.

Nutrition:

Calories: 61

Carbohydrates: 1g

Protein: .2g

Fat: .6g

Scrambled Eggs with Mushrooms and Cheese

Preparation Time: 10 minutes

Cooking Time: 20 minutes

Serving: 4

Ingredients:

- 4 tablespoons butter
- 8 eggs
- 4 tablespoons Parmesan cheese, shredded
- Salt and black pepper, to taste
- 1 cup fresh mushrooms, chopped finely

Directions:

1. Mix together eggs, salt, and black pepper in a bowl and beat well. Melt butter in a non-stick pan and add the beaten eggs. Cook for about 5 minutes and add Parmesan cheese and mushrooms. Cook for another 5 minutes, stirring occasionally. Let cool slightly and enjoy

Nutrition:

203 Calories

17.5g Fats

11.2g Proteins

Peanut Butter Chocolate Smoothie

Preparation Time: 5 minutes

Cooking Time: 0 minutes

Serving: 1

Ingredients:

- 1 tablespoon unsweetened cocoa powder
- 1 cup unsweetened coconut milk
- 1 tablespoon unsweetened peanut butter
- 1 pinch sea salt
- 5 drops stevia

Directions:

1. Mix all the ingredients until smooth. Pour into a glass and serve immediately.

Nutrition:

79 Calories

5.7g Fats

3.6g Proteins

Cream Cheese Pancakes

Preparation Time: 5 minutes

Cooking Time: 12 minutes

Serving: 4

Ingredients:

- 2 eggs
- ½ teaspoon cinnamon
- 2 oz. cream cheese
- 1 teaspoon granulated sugar substitute
- ½ cup almond flour

Directions:

1. Mix all the ingredients until smooth. Transfer the mixture into a medium bowl and put aside for about 3 minutes. Grease a large non-stick skillet with butter and add ¼ of mixture. Spread the mixture and cook until golden brown. Flip the pancake and let it cook. Do it again for the remaining mixture.

Nutrition:

170 Calories

4.3g Carbs

14.3g Fats

6.9g Proteins

Coconut Chia Pudding

Preparation Time: 10 minutes

Cooking Time: 25 minutes

Serving: 4

Ingredients:

- 1 cup full-fat coconut milk
- ¼ cup chia seeds
- ½ tablespoon honey
- 2 tablespoons almonds
- ¼ cup raspberries

Directions:

1. Mix together coconut milk, chia seeds, and honey in a bowl and refrigerate overnight.

Nutrition:

158 Calories

6.5g Carbs

14.1g Fats

2g Proteins

Morning Hash

Preparation Time: 10 minutes

Cooking Time: 30 minutes

Serving: 2

Ingredients:

- ½ teaspoon dried thyme, crushed
- ½ small onion, chopped
- 1 tablespoon butter
- ½ cup cauliflower florets, boiled
- ¼ cup heavy cream
- Salt and black pepper, to taste
- ½ pound cooked turkey meat, chopped

Directions:

1. Finely chop cauliflowers. Sauté butter and onion. Then add chopped cauliflower. Put turkey and let it cook. Mix in heavy cream and keep mixing it. Then serve.

Nutrition:

309 Calories

3.6g Carbs

34.3g Protein

17.1g Fat

Spanish Scramble

Preparation Time: 10 minutes

Cooking Time: 20 minutes

Serving: 2

Ingredients:

- 3 tablespoons butter
- 2 tablespoons scallions, sliced thinly
- 4 large organic eggs
- 1 Serrano chili pepper
- ¼ cup heavy cream
- 2 tablespoons cilantro, chopped finely
- 1 small tomato, chopped
- Salt and black pepper, to taste

Directions:

1. Mix cream, eggs, cilantro, salt and black pepper in a bowl. Sauté butter, tomatoes and Serrano pepper. Then add egg mixture and let it cook. Immediately serve it and topped with scallions

Nutrition:

180 Calories

2g Carbs

6.8g Protein

16.5g Fat

Cheese Waffles

Preparation Time: 10 minutes

Cooking Time: 20 minutes

Serving: 2

Ingredients:

- ½ cup Parmesan cheese, shredded
- 2 organic eggs, beaten
- 1 teaspoon onion powder
- 1 cup mozzarella cheese, shredded
- 1 tablespoon chives, minced
- ½ teaspoon ground black pepper
- 1 cup cauliflower
- 1 teaspoon garlic powder

Directions:

1. Mix all ingredients. Grease a waffle iron and heat it. Cook the mixture by batch until golden brown. Serve.

Nutrition:

149 Calories

6.1gCarbs

13.3g Protein

8.5g Fat

Spinach Frittata

Preparation Time: 20 minutes

Cooking Time: 45 minutes

Serving: 2

Ingredients:

- 1½ ounce dried bacon
- 2 ounces spinach, fresh
- 1½ ounce shredded cheese
- ½ tablespoon butter
- ¼ cup heavy whipped cream
- 2 eggs
- Salt and black pepper, to taste

Directions:

1. Grease and preheat oven at 360 degrees. Heat butter in a skillet and add bacon. Cook until crispy and add spinach. Stir thoroughly and keep aside. Mix eggs and cream. Then transfer it to the baking dish.

2. Add bacon spinach mixture to the baking dish and transfer to the oven. Bake for about 30 minutes and remove from the oven to serve.

Nutrition:

592 Calories

3.9g Carbs

39.1g Protein

46.7g Fat

Ketogenic Oatmeal

Preparation Time: 10 minutes

Cooking Time: 20 minutes

Serving: 2

Ingredients:

- 2 tablespoons flaxseeds
- 2 tablespoons sunflower seeds
- 2 cups coconut milk
- 2 tablespoons chia seeds
- 2 pinches of salt

Directions:

1. Mix all ingredients in a sauce pan. Let it simmer. Dish out in a bowl and serve warm.

Nutrition:

337 Calories

7.8g Carbs

4.9g Protein

32.6g Fat

Baked Eggs

Preparation Time: 5 minutes

Cooking Time: 10 minutes

Serving: 2

Ingredients:

- 2 eggs
- 3 ounces ground beef, cooked
- 2 ounces cheddar cheese, shredded

Directions:

1. Grease and preheat oven at 390 degrees. Arrange the cooked ground beef in a baking dish. Make two holes in the ground beef and crack eggs in them. Top with cheddar cheese and transfer the baking dish in the oven. Let it bake for 20 minutes. Allow it to cool for a bit and serve to enjoy. For meal prepping, you can refrigerate these baked eggs for about 2 days wrapped in a foil.

Nutrition:

512 Calories

1.4g Carbs

51g Protein

32.8g Fat

Blueberry Smoothie

Preparation Time: 5 minutes

Cooking Time: 15 minutes

Serving: 2

Ingredients:

- 1 cup fresh blueberries
- 1 teaspoon vanilla extract
- 28 ounces coconut milk
- 2 tablespoons lemon juice

Directions:

1. Blend all ingredients until smooth. Pour it in the glasses to serve and enjoy.

Nutrition:

152 Calories

6.9g Carbs

1.5g Protein

13.1g Fat

Quick Ketogenic Pancakes

Preparation Time: 15 minutes

Cooking Time: 30 minutes

Serving: 2

Ingredients:

- 3 ounces cottage cheese
- 2 eggs
- ½ tablespoon psyllium husk powder, ground
- ½ cup whipped cream
- 1 oz. butter

Directions:

1. Mix all ingredients except whipped cream and keep aside. Heat butter in the frying pan and pour half of the mixture. Cook it on each side and dish out in a serving platter. Add whipped cream in another bowl and whisk until smooth. Top the pancakes with whipped cream on them.

2. Meal Prep Tip: These Ketogenic pancakes can also be used as a snack. They taste awesome when serve cold.

Nutrition:

298 Calories

4.8g Carbs

12.2g Protein

26g Fat

Spinach Quiche

Preparation Time: 15 minutes

Cooking Time: 30 minutes

Serving: 2

Ingredients:

- 1½ cups Monterey Jack cheese, shredded
- ½ tablespoon butter, melted
- 5-ounce frozen spinach, thawed
- Salt and black pepper
- 2 eggs, beaten

Directions:

1. Grease and preheat the oven to 350 degrees. Heat butter on medium-low heat in a large skillet and add spinach. Cook for about 3 minutes and set aside. Mix together Monterey Jack cheese, eggs, spinach, salt and black pepper in a bowl.
2. Transfer the mixture into prepared pie dish and place in the oven. Bake for about 30 minutes serve by cutting into equal sized wedges.

Nutrition:

349 Calories

3.2g Carbs

23g Protein

27.8g Fat

Cream Crepes

Preparation Time: 15 minutes

Cooking Time: 25 minutes

Serving: 2

Ingredients:

- 1 teaspoon Splenda
- 2 tablespoons coconut flour
- 2 tablespoons coconut oil, melted and divided
- 2 organic eggs
- ½ cup heavy cream

Directions:

1. Put 1 tablespoon of coconut oil, eggs, Splenda and salt in a bowl and beat until well combined. Sift in the coconut flour slowly and beat constantly. Stir in the heavy cream and continuously beat until the mixture is well combined.

2. Put half mixture in a pan. Cook each side and repeat with the remaining mixture. Dish out to serve and enjoy. For meal prepping, wrap each cream crepe into wax paper pieces and place into a resealable bag. Freeze for up to 3 days and remove from the freezer. Microwave for about 2 minutes to serve.

Nutrition:

298 Calories

8g Carbs

7g Protein

27.1g Fat

Smoothie Bowl

Preparation Time: 5 minutes

Cooking Time: 0 minutes

Serving: 2

Ingredients:

- ¼ cup unsweetened almond milk
- 1 cup frozen strawberries
- ½ cup fat-free plain Greek yogurt
- 1 tablespoon walnuts, chopped
- ½ tablespoon unsweetened whey protein powder

Directions:

1. Blend strawberries until smooth. Add almond milk, Greek yogurt and whey protein powder in the blender and pulse for about 2 minutes. Transfer the mixture evenly into 2 bowls and top with walnuts to serve. You can wrap the bowls with plastic wrap and refrigerate for 2 days for meal prepping.

Nutrition:

71 Calories

19g Fat

6.3g Carbs

6.8g Protein

Almond Butter Muffins

Preparation Time: 10 minutes

Cooking Time: 25 minutes

Servings: 6

Ingredients:

- 1cups almond flour
- 1/2 cup powdered erythritol
- 1 teaspoons baking powder
- ¼ teaspoon salt
- ¾ cup almond butter, warmed
- ¾ cup unsweetened almond milk
- 2 large eggs

Directions:

1. Prepare oven to 350 ° F, and line a paper liner muffin pan.
2. In a mixing bowl, whisk the almond flour and the erythritol, baking powder, and salt.
3. Whisk the almond milk, almond butter, and the eggs together in a separate bowl.
4. Fill in wet ingredients into the dry until just mixed together.
5. Spoon the batter into the prepared pan and bake for 22 to 25 minutes until clean comes out the knife inserted in the middle.

6. Cook the muffins in the pan for 5 minutes. Then, switch onto a cooling rack with wire.

Nutrition:

135 Calories

11g Fat

6g Protein

Classic Western Omelet

Preparation Time: 5 minutes

Cooking Time: 10 minutes

Servings: 1

Ingredients:

- 2 teaspoons coconut oil
- 3 large eggs, whisked
- 1 tablespoon heavy cream
- Salt and pepper
- ¼ cup diced green pepper
- ¼ cup diced yellow onion
- ¼ cup diced ham

Directions:

1. Scourge eggs, heavy cream, salt, and pepper.
2. Heat up 1 teaspoon of coconut oil over medium heat in a small skillet.
3. Add the peppers and onions, then sauté the ham for 3 to 4 minutes.
4. Spoon the mixture in a cup, and heat the skillet with the remaining oil.
5. Mix in the whisked eggs and cook until the egg's bottom begins to set.
6. Tilt the pan and cook until almost set to spread the egg.

7. Spoon the ham and veggie mixture over half of the omelet and turn over.
8. Let cook the omelet until the eggs are set and then serve hot.

Nutrition:

415 Calories5

32.5g Fat

25g Protein

Sheet Pan Omelet

Preparation Time: 5 minutes

Cooking Time: 15 minutes

Servings: 6

Ingredients:

- 12 large eggs
- Salt and pepper
- 2 cups diced ham
- 1 cup shredded pepper jack cheese

Directions:

1. Prepare oven to 350°F and grease a rimmed baking sheet with cooking spray. Whisk the eggs in a mixing bowl then add salt and pepper until frothy. Stir in the ham and cheese. Pour the mixture in baking sheets and spread into an even layer. Bake for 13 minutes. Let cool slightly then cut it into squares to serve.

Nutrition:

235 Calories

15g Fat

21g Protein

Detoxifying Green Smoothie

Preparation Time: 5 minutes

Cooking Time: 0 minutes

Servings: 1

Ingredients:

- 1 cup fresh chopped kale
- ½ cup fresh baby spinach
- ¼ cup sliced celery
- 1 cup water
- 3 to 4 ice cubes
- 2 tablespoons fresh lemon juice
- 1 tablespoon fresh lime juice
- 1 tablespoon coconut oil
- Liquid stevia extract, to taste

Directions:

1. In a blender, add the broccoli, spinach, and celery. Stir in the rest of ingredients and blend until creamy. Pour into a big glass, and instantly enjoy it.

Nutrition:

160 Calories

14g Fat

2.5g Protein

Nutty Pumpkin Smoothie

Preparation Time: 5 minutes

Cooking Time: 0 minutes

Servings: 1

Ingredients:

- 1 cup unsweetened cashew milk
- ½ cup pumpkin puree
- ¼ cup heavy cream
- 1 tablespoon raw almonds
- ¼ teaspoon pumpkin pie spice
- Liquid stevia extract, to taste

Directions:

1. Incorporate all of the ingredients. Pulse the ingredients several times, then blend until creamy. Situate into a large glass and enjoy immediately.

Nutrition:

205 Calories

16.5g Fat

3g Protein

Salmon-Avocado Breakfast Boats

Preparation time: 10 minutes

Cooking time: 10 minutes

Servings: 4

Ingredients:

- 2 ripe avocados
- 4 ounces wild-caught smoked salmon
- 8 cherry tomatoes, halved
- 2 limes, for juice and garnish
- Sea salt and pepper to taste

Directions:

1. Marinate the salmon with lime juice for about an hour. Cut into thin strips and place into the avocado center. Top each avocado half with a lime wedge and several cherry tomato halves. Serve immediately.

Nutrition:

4g Carbohydrates

10g Protein

24g Total Fat

263 Calories

Buffalo Blue Cheese Omelet

Preparation time: 5 minutes

Cooking time: 10 minutes

Serving: 4

Ingredients:

- 4 ounces cream cheese, softened
- 4 tablespoons blue cheese
- 2 tablespoons hot sauce (adjust to suit your taste)
- 6 eggs
- 2 tablespoons water
- 2 tablespoons coconut oil
- Garnishes: Chopped fresh parsley and chives

Directions:

1. Heat the cream cheese, blue cheese, and hot sauce in the microwave for about 15 seconds. Stir until smooth and combined. Whisk eggs until foamy.
2. Heat about half a tablespoon of coconut oil in a non-stick pan over medium heat. Pour one quarter of the eggs into the pan. Drop one quarter of the cream cheese mixture by spoonful over half of the eggs.

3. Once the eggs have firmed up, fold the empty half over the half with filling. Let it cook for about another minute.
4. Carefully remove from pan, cover with tin foil to keep warm, and repeat with the remaining eggs and filling.

Nutrition:

2g Carbohydrates

12g Protein

26g Total Fat

282 Calories

Bacon, Egg & Cheese Fat Bombs

Preparation time: 10 minutes + 45 minutes refrigeration

Cooking time: 20 minutes

Servings: 5

Ingredients:

- 5 slices bacon
- 3 large eggs, hard boiled
- ¼ cup shredded cheddar cheese
- 1/3 cup butter, softened
- 3 tablespoons mayonnaise
- Sea salt and pepper to taste

Directions:

1. Preheat the oven to 375°F. Line a baking sheet with parchment paper. Lay the bacon flat and bake for 10–15 minutes until golden brown. Reserve any bacon grease for later use.
2. Peel and quarter the hard-boiled eggs. Mix egg and butter then mash well with a fork.
3. Stir in the shredded cheese, mayonnaise and any leftover bacon grease. Season with salt and pepper. Mix well and let it chill until firm.
4. Remove the egg mixture from the refrigerator and form into 5 balls. Wrap each ball in a slice

bacon and store in an airtight container until ready to serve.

Nutrition:

2g Carbohydrates

8g Protein

28g Total Fat

292 Calories

Cheesy Scrambled Eggs & Greens

Preparation time: 5 minutes

Cooking time: 10 minutes

Serving: 4

Ingredients:

- 8 large eggs
- 6 cups kale, baby spinach, or Swiss Chard
- 1 cup shredded mozzarella cheese
- 2 tablespoons olive oil
- 2 tablespoons heavy cream
- Sea salt and pepper to taste
- Optional: Meat lovers add some bacon and/or sausage while cooking the spinach, or for a non-meat option, top with half a sliced avocado.

Directions:

1. Crack the eggs into a medium bowl. Add the heavy cream to the eggs and season with salt and pepper. Whisk until well combined. Roughly chop your greens.
2. Heat the olive oil. Add the baby spinach to the pan. Stir frequently, being careful not to burn.

Once the spinach has wilted, reduce heat to low.

3. Add egg to the spinach and slowly stir until the eggs are almost set. Add the cheddar cheese and stir until well combined. Once the cheese has melted, divide onto four plates and serve!

Nutrition:

6g Carbohydrates

16g Protein

19g Total Fat

251 Calories

Mocha-Coconut Chia Pudding

Preparation time: 5 minutes + 30 minutes refrigeration

Cooking time: 10 minutes

Servings: 4

Ingredients:

- 4 tablespoons instant coffee
- 2 tablespoons cocoa powder
- ½ cup chia seeds
- ½ cup coconut cream
- 1 tablespoon vanilla extract
- 2 tablespoons sugar substitute
- 4 tablespoons cacao nibs
- 2 cups water

Directions:

1. Prepare a strong cup of coffee by simmering the instant coffee with 2 cups of water until the liquid is about 1 cup. Whisk the cocoa powder, coconut cream, vanilla extract, and sugar substitute into the coffee.

2. Mix in the chia seeds and cacao nibs. Mix well. Divide into 4 small serving dishes and allow to set for at least 30 minutes. Remove from refrigerator, garnish with a few additional cacao nibs, and serve!

Nutrition:

14g Carbohydrates

7g Protein

11g Fat

257 Calories

Pumpkin Muffins

Preparation time: 10 minutes

Cooking time: 30 minutes

Serving: 6

Ingredients:

- 2/3 cup pumpkin puree
- 1 ½ cups almond flour
- 1 tablespoon pumpkin pie spice mix
- 2/3 cup sugar substitute
- 4 large eggs
- 1 teaspoon baking powder

Directions:

1. Line the muffin pan and preheat oven to 300°F. In a large bowl, combine the almond flour, pumpkin pie spice, and sugar substitute. Mix well.
2. Add the pumpkin puree and eggs. Beat with an electric mixer until smooth. Evenly divide the batter among the 6 paper liners and bake until a toothpick inserted into the middle of a muffin comes out clean.
3. Let it cool. Transfer in an airtight container until ready to serve.

Nutrition:

9g Carbohydrates:

9g Protein

13g Total Fat

168 Calories

Almond Flour Pancakes

Preparation time: 10 minutes

Cooking time: 5–10 minutes

Serving: 4

Ingredients:

- 1 cup almond flour
- 4 large eggs
- ¼ cup coconut oil, melted
- 1 teaspoon vanilla extract
- ¼ cup sugar substitute
- ½ teaspoon baking soda
- 1 teaspoon cream of tartar
- ¼ cup full-fat, plain yogurt
- ½ cup fresh blueberries
- Additional coconut oil to grease the pan

Directions:

1. Whisk the eggs until frothy. Mix together the almond flour, sugar substitute, baking soda, and cream of tartar until well combined.

2. Stir the vanilla extract and the melted coconut oil into the eggs. Add the dry ingredients to the wet and mix well. Drizzle with water if the mixture seems too thick (it should be a bit thicker than regular pancake batter).

3. Grease a large skillet with about a teaspoon of coconut oil and spoon or ladle 2–3 small pancakes for every serving. Cook on medium-low for about 5 minutes until the pancake starts to firm up. Flip and cook the other side for about a minute.
4. Remove from skillet, keep it warm with foil and repeat with remaining pancake batter. Top each serving of pancakes with yogurt and berries. Serve and enjoy!

Nutrition:

9g Carbohydrates

12g Protein

33g Total Fat

368 Calories

Warm Grain-Free Cereal

Preparation time: 5 minutes

Cooking time: 8 minutes

Serving: 4

Ingredients:

- 1 1/3 cup crushed walnut pieces
- 1 1/3 cup sliced almonds, chopped
- 1 1/3 cup macadamia nut pieces, toasted
- 1 1/3 cup flaxseeds
- 1 1/3 cup hemp hearts
- 1 1/3 cup chia seeds
- 1 1/3 cup chopped cashews
- 6 tablespoons butter
- 1 cup unsweetened, shredded coconut
- 4 cups unsweetened almond milk
- Liquid stevia to taste (if desired)
- Pinch of salt

Directions:

1. Preheat oven to 250°F. Toast the nuts and shredded coconut (keep separate from each other) until golden brown. In a saucepan over medium heat, melt the butter.
2. Add the toasted nuts and a pinch of salt. Let cook for 1–2 minutes, stirring constantly. Add

the toasted coconut and continue stirring. Add the milk and liquid stevia, if using. Allow to cook for 5–7 minutes, until heated throughout. Remove from heat, divide into 4 bowls and serve immediately.

Nutrition:

10g Carbohydrates

9g Protein

62g Total Fat

603 Calories

Corned Beef Hash and Eggs

Preparation time: 3 minutes

Cooking time: 12 minutes

Serving: 4

Ingredients:

- 2 cups cooked corned beef, chopped
- 4 large eggs
- 1 small yellow onion, diced
- 1-pound parsnips, peeled and diced
- 2 cloves garlic, minced
- ½ cup beef or chicken broth
- 2 tablespoons olive oil
- Sea salt and pepper to taste

Directions:

1. Heat olive oil. Sauté onion and garlic.
2. Add the parsnips and let it cook. Reduce heat to medium-low, pour in the beef broth, cover and cook until the parsnips are tender and the liquid has been absorbed.
3. Add the chopped corned beef and stir until well combined. On top of the hash, put the eggs season with salt and pepper, cover, and continue cooking for 5–7 minutes, or until eggs

are cooked to your desired level of doneness. Serve immediately.

Nutrition:

14g Carbohydrates

23g Protein

26g Total Fat

416 Calories

Spiced Pear Breakfast Bars

Preparation time: 5 minutes

Cooking time: 22 minutes

Serving: 6

Ingredients:

- 1 large pear, cored and peeled
- 3 large eggs
- 2 tablespoons coconut oil
- 2 tablespoons maple syrup
- ¼ cup coconut flour
- 1 teaspoon cinnamon
- ½ teaspoon nutmeg
- ¼ teaspoon cloves
- ½ teaspoon baking soda
- ¼ teaspoon salt

Directions:

1. Line and preheat oven to 350°F. In a food processor, pulse the apple until pureed. Mix eggs, maple syrup, and coconut oil. Blend until well combined.

2. Mix salt, baking soda, cinnamon, nutmeg, cloves, and coconut flour. Mix until just combined. Pour the batter into the prepared

pan. Sprinkle with additional cinnamon, if desired.

3. Bake until a toothpick inserted comes out clean. Allow to cool on a wire rack. Cut into 6 squares.

Nutrition:

10g Carbohydrates

4g Protein

9g Total Fat:

127 Calories

Scrambled Eggs with Buttered Basil

Preparation Time: 5 minutes

Cooking Time: 15 minutes

Servings: 2

Ingredients:

- 2 ounces butter
- 4 eggs
- 4 tbsp. coconut cream or coconut milk or sour cream
- 4 tbsp. fresh basil
- Salt to taste

Directions:

1. Situate non-stick pan on low heat and melt butter. In a small bowl, whisk eggs, coconut cream, basil and salt. Pour into hot pan. With a spatula, stir eggs until scrambled and cooked to desired doneness. Serve warm, or place in meal prep container to save for later.

Nutrition:

427 Calories

42g Fat

13g Protein

Breakfast Bake

Preparation Time: 10 minutes

Cooking Time: 50 minutes

Servings: 8

Ingredients:

- 1 tbsp. olive oil
- 1-pound sausage
- 8 large eggs
- 2 cups cooked spaghetti squash
- 1 tbsp. chopped fresh oregano
- Sea salt
- Freshly ground black pepper
- ½ cup shredded Cheddar cheese

Directions:

1. Preheat the oven to 375. Slightly grease a 9-by-13-inch casserole dish using olive oil and set aside. Place a large ovenproof skillet over medium-heat and add the olive oil.
2. Brown the sausage until cooked through, about 5 minutes. While the sausage is cooking, whisk together the eggs, squash, and oregano in a medium bowl. Season lightly and set aside.

3. Mix in cooked sausage to the egg mixture, stir until just combined, and pour the mixture into the casserole dish.

4. Garnish top of the casserole with the cheese and cover the casserole loosely with aluminum foil.

5. Bake the casserole for 30 minutes, and then remove the foil and bake for another 15 minutes.

6. Set aside for 10 minutes before serving

Nutrition:

303 Calories

24g Fat

17g Protein

Nutty Granola

Preparation Time: 10 minutes

Cooking Time: 1 hour

Serving: 8

Ingredients:

- 2 cups shredded unsweetened coconut
- 1 cup sliced almonds
- 1 cup raw sunflower seeds
- ½ cup raw pumpkin seeds
- ½ cup walnuts
- ½ cup melted coconut oil
- 10 drips liquid Stevia
- 1 tsp. ground cinnamon
- ½ tsp. ground nutmeg

Direction:

1. Preheat the oven to 250 degrees. Line 2 baking sheets with parchment paper. Set aside. Throw together the shredded coconut, almonds, sunflower seeds, pumpkin seeds, and walnuts in a large bowl until mixed.

2. In a small bowl, scourge the coconut oil, stevia, cinnamon, and nutmeg until blended. Fill the coconut oil mixture into the nut mixture and use your hands to blend.

3. Spread granola mixture to the baking sheets and spread it out evenly. Bake the granola for 1 hour.
4. Situate granola to a large bowl and let the granola cool, tossing it frequently to break up the large pieces.

Nutrition:

391 Calories

38g Fat

10g Protein

Nutty Blueberry Muffins

Preparation Time: 10 minutes

Cooking Time: 17 minutes

Serving: 10

Ingredients:

- 2 eggs
- 1 cup fresh blueberries
- ¼ cup Flaxseed Meal
- ½ cup Almond slices
- 1 tbsp. almond butter
- ½ cup Unsweetened almond milk
- 1 cup almond flour
- 1 tbsp. baking powder
- 2 tbsp. butter (melted)
- 1 tbsp. Olive oil
- 1/3 cup Sweetener
- 1 tsp. Vanilla extract

Directions:

1. While prepping the oven to 350°F, scourge 2 eggs and sweetener in a mixing bowl for around 5 minutes.

2. Put the baking powder, almond four, almond butter, almond milk, and the flaxseed meal in the egg mixture. Then pour the melted butter,

the vanilla extract, and the olive oil. Stir the ingredients together. Gently drop the shaved almonds and fresh blueberries into the mixture and fold.

3. Prepare a muffin or cupcake pan and transfer the batter into it. Top with additional shaved almonds. Bake for 17 minutes.

4. Remove from the oven and enjoy.

Nutrition:

167 Calories

14g Fat

5.6g Protein

Low-Carb Pancakes

Preparation Time 5 minutes

Cooking Time 5 minutes

Servings: 12

Ingredients:

- 3 tbsp. coconut flour
- 3 tbsp. sour cream
- ¼ cup butter softened
- 4 eggs
- 1 tsp. baking powder
- 1 tsp. vanilla extract
- 1 tbsp. powdered sweetener
- ¼ cup water

Directions:

1. Incorporate all dry ingredients in a medium-sized bowl. Mix well and set aside. In a large mixing bowl, combine sour cream with butter, vanilla extract, and water. Mix on high for 2 minutes. Stir eggs, one at a time, beating constantly.

2. Add dry ingredients and continue to mix for 3 minutes. Grease a non-stick skillet with oil and heat over medium-high heat. Using a large

spoon, pour batter into skillet and cook for 2 minutes. Flip and continue cooking.

3. Serve immediately.

Nutrition:

78 Calories

2.5g Protein

1.5g Carbs

Avocado and Eggs

Preparation Time: 10 minutes

Cooking Time: 20 minutes

Servings: 4

Ingredients

- 2 avocados, peeled, halved lengthwise
- 4 large eggs
- 1 (4 oz.) chicken breast, cooked and shredded
- ¼ cup Cheddar cheese
- Sea salt
- Freshly ground pepper

Directions:

1. Prep the oven to 425°F. Take a spoon and scrape out each side of the avocado halves until the hole is about twice the original size.

2. Position the avocado halves in an 8-by-8-inch baking dish, hollow side up. Crack an egg into each hollow and divide the shredded chicken between each avocado half. Sprinkle the cheese on top of each and season lightly with the salt and pepper.

3. Bake the avocados for 20 minutes. Serve immediately.

Nutrition:

324 Calories

25g Fat

19g Protein

Mushroom Frittata

Preparation Time: 10 minutes

Cooking Time: 15 minutes

Serving: 6

Ingredients:

- 2 tbsp. olive oil
- 1 cup sliced fresh mushrooms
- 1 cup shredded spinach
- 6 bacon slices, cooked and chopped
- 10 large eggs, beaten
- ½ cup crumbled goat cheese
- Sea salt
- Freshly ground black pepper

Directions:

1. Preheat the oven to 350°F. Situate big ovenproof skillet over medium-high heat and add the olive oil. Sauté the mushrooms until lightly browned, about 3 minutes.

2. Add the spinach and bacon and sauté until the greens are wilted, about 1 minute. Add the eggs and cook, lifting the edges of the frittata with a spatula so uncooked egg flow underneath, for 3 to 4 minutes.

3. Sprinkle the top with the crumbled goat cheese and season lightly with salt and pepper. Bake until set and lightly browned, about 15 minutes. Remove the frittata from the oven, and let stand for 5 minutes.

4. Cut into 6 wedges and serve immediately.

Nutrition:

316 Calories

27g Fat

16g Protein

Artichoke Omelet

Preparation Time: 10 minutes

Cooking Time: 10 minutes

Serving: 4

Ingredients:

- 6 eggs, beaten
- 2 tbsp. heavy(whipping) cream
- 8 bacon slices, cooked and chopped
- 1 tbsp. olive oil
- ¼ cup chopped onion
- ½ cup chopped artichoke hearts (canned, packed in water)
- Sea Salt
- Freshly ground black pepper

Directions:

1. In a small bowl, scourge the eggs, heavy cream, and bacon until well blended and set aside. Situate skillet over medium-high heat and add the olive oil.
2. Sauté the onion until tender, about 3 minutes. Pour the mixture into the skillet, swirling it for 1 minute.
3. Cook the omelet, lifting the edges with a spatula to let the uncooked egg flow

underneath, for 2 minutes. Sprinkle the artichoke hearts on top and flip the omelet. Cook for 4 minutes more, until the egg is firm. Flip the omelet over again so the artichoke hearts area on top.

4. Remove from the heat, cut the omelet into quarters, and season with salt and black pepper. Serve while hot.

Nutrition:

435 Calories

39g Fat

17g Protein

Low-Carb Crepe

Preparation Time: 5 minutes

Cooking Time: 10 minutes

Servings 2

Ingredients:

- Batter
- 2 oz. cream cheese (full fat)
- 2 eggs

Topping

- ½ cup mixed berries
- 2 tsp. heavy whipping cream

Direction:

1. Melt cream cheese in a microwave. Stir in 2 eggs to cream cheese (one at a time) and mix well. Use a hand blender or a whisk. Add any spices to the mixture (optional). Warm up a skillet, oil it slightly and make your crepes.

Nutrition:

162 Calories

14.2g Fat

7.7g Protein

Cinnamon Almond Butter Smoothie

Preparation Time 5 minutes

Cooking Time 2 minutes

Servings: 1

Ingredients:

- 1 ½ cups unsweetened nut milk
- 1 scoop collagen peptides
- 2 tbsp. almond butter
- ½ tsp. cinnamon
- 15 drops liquid stevia
- 1/8 tsp. almond extract
- 1/8 tsp. salt
- 6-8 ice cubes

Direction:

1. Incorporate all the ingredients to a blender and combine for 30 seconds or until you get a smooth consistency.

Nutrition:

326 Calories

27g Fats

19g Protein

Kale Wrapped Eggs

Preparation Time: 8-10 minutes

Cooking Time: 5 minutes

Servings: 4

Ingredients:

- Three tablespoons heavy cream
- Four hardboiled eggs
- ¼ teaspoon pepper
- Four kale leaves
- Four prosciutto slices
- ¼ teaspoon salt
- 1 ½ cups water

Directions:

1. Peel the eggs and wrap each with the kale. Wrap them in the prosciutto slices and sprinkle with ground black pepper and salt. Place it in your instant pot and pour water. Arrange the eggs over the trivet/basket.

2. Close the lid and lock it. Press "MANUAL" cooking function; timer to 5 minutes with default "HIGH" pressure mode. Allow the pressure to build to cook. After cooking time is over press "CANCEL" setting. Find and press

"QPR" cooking function. This setting is for quick release of inside pressure.

3. Slowly open and take it out from the lid.

Nutrition:

247 Calories

20g Fat

19g Protein

Zucchini Ketogenic Bread

Preparation Time: 8-10 minutes

Cooking Time: 40 minutes

Servings: 12-16 slices

Ingredients:

- 1 cup grated zucchini
- 2 ½ cups almond flour
- ½ cup chopped walnuts
- 3 eggs
- ½ cup olive oil
- 1 ½ teaspoon baking powder
- Pinch of ginger powder
- 1 teaspoon vanilla extract
- ½ teaspoon cinnamon
- ¼ teaspoon nutmeg
- pinch of sea salt
- 1 ½ cups water

Directions:

1. Whisk together the wet ingredients in a bowl. Combine the dry ingredients in another bowl. Combine the dry and wet mixture. Stir in the zucchini.
2. Grease a loaf pan and pour the mixture. Top with chopped walnuts. Open its top lid and pour

water. Arrange a trivet or steamer basket inside that came with Instant Pot. Now arrange the loaf pan over the trivet/basket.

3. Close the lid and press "MANUAL" cooking function; timer to 40 minutes with default "HIGH" pressure mode. Allow the pressure to build to cook the ingredients. After cooking time is over press "CANCEL" setting. Find and press "QPR" cooking function. This setting is for quick release of inside pressure.

4. Slowly open the lid, take out the cooked bread. Cool down, slice, and serve.

Nutrition:

164 Calories

17g Fat

5g Protein

Ham Sausage Quiche

Preparation Time: 8-10 minutes

Cooking Time: 30 minutes

Servings: 4

Ingredients:

- 4 bacon slices, cooked and crumbled
- ½ cup diced ham
- 2 green onions, chopped
- ½ cup full-fat milk
- Six eggs, beaten
- 1 cup ground sausage, cooked
- 1 cup shredded cheddar cheese
- ¼ teaspoon salt
- Pinch of pepper
- 1 ½ cups water

Directions:

1. Grease a baking dish with coconut oil cooking spray. Place all of the ingredients in a bowl, and stir to combine. Add this mixture to the prepared dish.

2. Open its top lid and pour water. Arrange a trivet or steamer basket inside that came with Instant Pot. Now arrange the dish over the trivet/basket.

3. Close the lid and press "MANUAL" cooking function; timer to 30 minutes with default "HIGH" pressure mode. Allow the pressure to build to cook. After cooking time is over press "CANCEL" setting. Find and press "QPR" cooking function. This setting is for quick release of inside pressure.

4. Place the dish on the rack in your IP and close the lid. Cook on high and release the pressure naturally. Slowly open the lid, take out the cooked recipe in serving plates or serving bowls, and enjoy the Ketogenic recipe.

Nutrition:

398 Calories

31g Fat

26g Protein

Coconut Almond Breakfast

Preparation Time: 8-10 minutes

Cooking Time: 5 minutes

Servings: 2

Ingredients:

- 2 tablespoons roasted pepitas
- 1/3 cup coconut milk
- 2 tablespoon chopped almonds
- 1 tablespoon chia seeds
- 1/3 cup water
- One handful blueberries

Directions:

1. Mix the pepitas with almonds and blend well. Switch on the pot. Add the chia seeds with water and coconut milk; gently stir to mix well. Add the pepita mix and combine.

2. Close the lid and press "MANUAL" cooking function; timer to 5 minutes with default "HIGH" pressure mode. Allow the pressure to cook.

3. After cooking time is over press "CANCEL" setting. Find and press "QPR" cooking function. This setting is for quick release of inside

pressure. Slowly open and take out the dish from the lid.

Nutrition:

148 Calories

6g Fat

2g Protein

Avocado Egg Muffins

Preparation Time: 8-10 minutes

Cooking Time: 12 minutes

Servings: 4

Ingredients:

- 1 ½ cups of coconut milk
- 2 avocados, diced
- 4 ½ ounces (grated or shredded) cheese
- ½ cup almond flour
- 5 bacon slices, cooked and crumbled
- 5 eggs, beaten
- 2 tablespoon butter
- 3 spring onions, diced
- 1 teaspoon oregano
- ¼ cup flaxseed meal
- 1 ½ tablespoon lemon juice
- 1 teaspoon minced garlic
- 1 teaspoon onion powder
- 1 teaspoon salt
- Pinch of pepper
- 1 teaspoon baking powder
- 1 ½ cups water

Directions:

1. Whisk together the wet ingredients. Stir in the dry ingredients gradually until turns smooth. Stir in the avocado, bacon, onions, and cheese. Add the mixture into 16 muffin cups. Arrange Instant Pot over a dry platform in your kitchen. Open its top lid and switch it on.

2. In the pot, pour water. Arrange the 8 cups over the trivet/basket.

3. Close the lid and press "MANUAL" cooking function; timer to 12 minutes with default "HIGH" pressure mode. Allow the pressure to cook.

4. After cooking time is over press "CANCEL" setting. Find and press "QPR" cooking function. This setting is for quick release of inside pressure. Slowly open and take out the dish from the pot.

5. Repeat the same process.

Nutrition:

146 Calories

11g Fat

6g Protein

Soft-Boiled Eggs

Preparation Time: 5 minutes

Cooking Time: 3 minutes

Servings: 4

Ingredients:

- 4 Eggs
- 2 cups Water

Directions:

1. Switch on the instant pot, pour in water, insert steamer basket and place eggs in it.
2. Shut the instant pot with its lid in the sealed position, then press the 'manual' button, press '+/-' to set the cooking time to 3 minutes and cook at low-pressure setting; when the pressure builds in the pot, the cooking timer will start.
3. When the instant pot buzzes, press the 'keep warm' button, do a quick pressure release and open the lid.
4. Fill a bowl with ice water, place eggs in it from the instant pot, and let rest for 3 minutes.
5. Then peel the eggs, cut into slices, season with salt and black pepper and serve.

Nutrition:

68 Calories

4.6g Fat

5.5g Protein

Breakfast Casserole

Preparation Time: 10 minutes

Cooking Time: 45 minutes

Servings: 6

Ingredients:

- 1/2 teaspoon salt
- 2 tablespoons avocado oil
- 6 ounces breakfast sausage
- 1 1/2 cups Broccoli stalks, grated
- 1 tablespoon Minced garlic
- ½ teaspoon Ground black pepper
- 6 eggs
- 1/4 cup Heavy cream
- 1 cup Monterey jack cheese, grated
- 1 cup Water
- 1 Green onion sliced
- 1 California avocado, sliced
- ¼ cup Sour cream

Directions:

1. Switch on the instant pot, grease the pot with oil, press the 'sauté/simmer' button, and add the sausage and cook until the meat is no longer pink.

2. Then add broccoli along with garlic, season with salt and black pepper and continue cooking for 2 minutes.

3. Take a 7-inch baking dish, grease it with oil, spoon in cooked broccoli mixture and spread evenly.

4. Crack the eggs in a bowl, add cream, whisk until combined, and then add onion and cheese, whisk until mixed, pour the mixture over the sausage mixture and cover with aluminum foil.

5. Press the 'keep warm' button, wipe the instant pot clean, pour in water, then insert trivet stand and place baking dish on it.

6. Shut the instant pot with its lid in the sealed position, then press the 'manual' button, press '+/-' to set the cooking time to 35 minutes and cook at high-pressure setting; when the pressure builds in the pot, the cooking timer will start.

7. When the instant pot buzzes, press the 'keep warm' button, release pressure naturally for 10 minutes, then do quick pressure release and open the lid.

8. Take out the baking dish, uncover it and turn it over the plate to take out the frittata.
9. Top the frittata with avocado, cut into slices and the top with sour cream.

Nutrition:

351 Calories

28.5g Fat

18.6g Protein

Poblano Cheese Frittata

Preparation Time: 5 minutes

Cooking Time: 35 minutes

Servings: 4

Ingredients:

- 4 Eggs
- 10 oz. Diced green chili
- 1 tsp. Salt
- ½ tsp. Ground cumin
- 1 cup Mexican cheese blend, shredded, divided
- ¼ cup Chopped cilantro
- 2 cups Water

Directions:

1. Crack eggs in a bowl, add green chilies, half-and-half, and ½ cup cheese, season with salt and cumin, stir well until incorporated. Take a 6-inch baking dish or silicone pan, grease it with oil, pour in the egg mixture and cover with aluminum foil.

2. Switch on the instant pot, pour water in it, then insert trivet stand and place baking dish on it. Shut the instant pot with its lid in the sealed position, then press the 'manual' button, press '+/-' to set the cooking time to 20 minutes and

cook at high-pressure setting; when the pressure builds in the pot, the cooking timer will start.

3. When the instant pot buzzes, press the 'keep warm' button, release pressure naturally for 10 minutes, then do a quick pressure release and open the lid. Meanwhile, switch on the broiler and let it preheat.

4. Take out the baking dish, spread remaining cheese on top, then place it under the broiler and broil for 5 minutes or until cheese melts and the top is nicely browned.

5. When done, turn the dish over a plate to take out the frittata, then cut into slices and serve.

Nutrition:

257 Calories

19g Fat

14g Protein

Poached Egg

Preparation Time: 5 minutes

Cooking Time: 7 minutes

Servings: 4

Ingredients:

- ¾ teaspoon salt
- ¾ teaspoon ground black pepper
- 1 cup water
- 4 eggs

Directions:

1. Take a silicone tray, grease it with avocado oil and then crack the eggs into the cups of the tray. Switch on the instant pot, pour water in it, insert a trivet stand and place the silicone tray on it.

2. Shut the instant pot with its lid in the sealed position, then press the 'manual' button, press '+/-' to set the cooking time to 7 minutes and cook at high-pressure setting; when the pressure builds in the pot, the cooking timer will start.

3. When the instant pot buzzes, press the 'keep warm' button, do a quick pressure release and open the lid. Ensure all eggs are cooked; egg

whites should be firm, and yolk should be slightly jiggled.

4. Run a knife around each cup in the tray, then gently scoop out the egg and transfer to a serving plate. Season poached eggs with salt and black pepper and serve straight away.

Nutrition:

72 Calories

4.8g Fat

6.3g Protein

Spinach Egg Bites

Preparation Time: 5 minutes

Cooking Time: 20 minutes

Servings: 7

Ingredients:

- 4 Eggs
- ¾ cup Parmesan cheese, grated
- ¼ cup Heavy whipping cream
- ¼ cup Spinach, chopped
- ½ oz. Prosciutto, chopped
- ½ tsp. Ground black pepper
- 1/8 tsp. Salt
- 1 ½ cup Water

Directions:

1. Take an egg bite mold tray having seven cups and fill the cups evenly with prosciutto and spinach. Crack eggs in a bowl, add remaining ingredients except for water and whisk until smooth.

2. Switch on the instant pot, pour in water and place trivet stand in it. Pour egg mixture evenly over spinach and prosciutto, 4 tablespoons per cup or more until 3/4th filled, and then cover the pan with aluminum foil.

3. Place pan on the trivet stand, shut the instant pot with its lid in the sealed position, then press the 'manual' button, press '+/-' to set the cooking time to 10 minutes and cook at high-pressure setting; when the pressure builds in the pot, the cooking timer will start.

4. When the instant pot buzzes, press the 'keep warm' button, release pressure naturally for 10 minutes, then do a quick pressure release and open the lid.

5. Take out the tray, uncover it and turn over the pan onto a plate to take out the egg bites. Serve straight away.

Nutrition:

400 Calories

29g Fat

27g Protein

Bacon Cheeseburger Waffles

Preparation Time: 10 minutes

Cooking Time: 20 minutes

Servings: 4

Ingredients

Toppings

- Pepper and Salt to taste
- 12 ounces of cheddar cheese
- 4 tablespoons of sugar-free barbecue sauce
- 4 slices of bacon
- 4 ounces of ground beef, 70% lean meat and 30% fat

Waffle dough

- Pepper and salt to taste
- 3 tablespoons of parmesan cheese, grated
- 4 tablespoons of almond flour
- ¼ teaspoon of onion powder
- ¼ teaspoon of garlic powder
- 1 cup (125 g) of cauliflower crumbles
- 2 large eggs
- ounces of cheddar cheese

Directions

1. Shred about 3 ounces of cheddar cheese, then add in cauliflower crumbles in a bowl and put in half of the cheddar cheese.
2. Put into the mixture spices, almond flour, eggs, and parmesan cheese, then mix and put aside for some time.
3. Thinly cut the bacon and cook in a skillet on medium to high heat.
4. After the bacon is cooked partially, put in the beef, cook until the mixture is well done.
5. Then put the excess grease from the bacon mixture into the waffle mixture. Set aside the bacon mix.
6. Use an immersion blender to blend the waffle mix until it becomes a paste, then add into the waffle iron half of the mix and cook until it becomes crispy.
7. Repeat for the remaining waffle mixture.
8. As the waffles cook, add sugar-free barbecue sauce to the ground beef and bacon mixture in the skillet.
9. Then proceed to assemble waffles by topping them with half of the left cheddar cheese and half the beef mixture. Repeat this for the

remaining waffles, broil for around 1-2 minutes until the cheese has melted then serve right away.

Nutrition:

18.8g Protein

33.9g Fats

415 Calories

Ketogenic Breakfast Cheesecake

Preparation Time: 20 minutes

Cooking Time: 45 minutes

Servings: 24

Ingredients

Toppings

- 1/4 cup of mixed berries for each cheesecake, frozen and thawed
- Filling ingredients
- 1/2 teaspoon of vanilla extract
- 1/2 teaspoon of almond extract
- 3/4 cup of sweetener
- 6 eggs
- 8 ounces of cream cheese
- 16 ounces of cottage cheese

Crust ingredients

- 4 tablespoons of salted butter
- 2 tablespoons of sweetener
- 2 cups of almonds, whole

Directions

1. Preheat oven to around 350 degrees F.
2. Pulse almonds in a food processor then add in butter and sweetener.

3. Pulse until all the ingredients mix well and coarse dough forms.
4. Coat twelve silicone muffin pans using foil or paper liners.
5. Portion the batter evenly between the muffin pans then press into the bottom part until it forms a crust and bakes for about 8 minutes.
6. Pulse in a food processor the cream cheese and cottage cheese then pulse until the mixture is smooth.
7. Put in the extracts and sweetener then combine until well mixed.
8. Add in eggs and pulse again until it becomes smooth. Share equally the batter between the muffin pans, then bake for around 30-40 minutes.
9. Put aside until cooled completely, then put in the refrigerator for about 2 hours and then top with frozen and thawed berries.

Nutrition

12g Fats

152 Calories

6g Proteins